Quick Knowledge....How to get rid of Belly Fat. What to eat & what to avoid.
By Manal Mano

Table of Contents

Introduction

Getting rid of your belly fat is important for more than just vanity's sake. Belly fat not only looks undesirable, it is also documented to have dangerous health implications.

According to Harvard Medical School the visceral fat stored in your midsection is "biologically active". In fact, experts think of it more like an extra organ or gland because it produces hormones that can affect your health, especially those related to appetite and metabolism, like adiponectin and leptin.

Latest research links belly fat to everything from heart disease and type 2 diabetes to certain cancers and even an increased risk of dementia. Belly fat is associated with breast cancer, asthma, cardiovascular diseases and problems with functions of reproductive systems.

Fortunately, reducing your belly fat is as simple as adopting a healthier lifestyle. By practicing regular exercises and introducing healthy foods into your diet is enough to boost your immune system to transform your body and mind.

This short ebook aims to give you a quick affective knowledge on how to lose belly fat. Within just 45 minutes you will have gained some essential knowledge to make a difference to your life right now. You will learn the reasons for belly fat, the foods you need to avoid, the foods that fight belly fat for that perfect flat stomach.

This book provides you with a guide to the smoothie diet; a popular fast and easy nutritious option. You will also learn how you can still enjoy your favorite meals whilst maintaining a body fat loss diet with the 5:2 Fast diet.

The Cause of Belly Fat

Eating When Sad, Angry or Upset
Emotional eating is eating whenever you're upset or stressed out as a way to ease or disguise the pain. There is no conscious thought involved, and in truth, does nothing other than build hideous belly fat. Instead, when in a stressful situation you should drink a glass of water, talk to a friend, or take a relaxing walk. Choose an activity that doesn't involve eating, so you can stop yourself from loading up on extra calories when you're feeling emotional.

Drinking Carbonated Soda Drinks Regularly
According to researchers, consuming one or two cans of soda daily causes your waistline to increase at least five times faster than those who rarely drink soda in the course of a week. The high amount of sugar used in sodas triggers your craving for food, so you end up eating more than you should during mealtimes. And don't be fooled by diet sodas which contain artificial sweeteners, and can increase your appetite as much as sugar does. So when you have that serious craving for a refreshing drink, opt for healthy smoothies, fresh fruit juices, or a glass of water with lemon zest and mint leaves.

Consuming Low-Fat Foods More Often

Be wary of too many low-fat foods, since manufacturers often add sugar to these items and the more sugar you have in the body, the greater your chances of storing more body fat. There is an assumption that high-fat foods and drinks lead to more fat storage in your belly. The truth is, monounsaturated fats are not bad for you. If anything, foods such as avocados, olive oil and seeds work well in eliminating belly fat.

Insufficient Protein in Your Regular Diet

Have you been depriving your body of protein-rich foods? Generally, healthy adults should consume at least 20 to 25 grams of protein in each meal, although this depends on your activity level and body size.

To power up your daily meals, consider eating low fat and high protein content foods such as ricotta cheese, shellfish, turkey, skinless chicken, salmon and eggs.

Using a Large Plate

The size of the plate you use has a direct effect on the volume of food you eat. In a survey conducted among obese individuals, it was discovered that these people prefer larger plates over smaller or medium-sized ones. When you have a larger plate with more empty space to pile up your food, you tend to consume more than your body needs, and that leads to more fat stored in your body. The simple choice to use a smaller plate to eat from can have a substantial impact on your life.

Depriving Yourself of Sleep

Adults should get about seven to nine hours of sleep each night to properly rest and replenish the body. When you fail to get enough sleep, your level of the stress hormone Cortisol increases and causes you to crave sugary foods. With that in mind, it becomes harder to get rid of belly fat when you are in the habit of not getting enough regular sleep. To maintain normal levels of cortisol, try your best to attain the recommended hours of sleep every night. This way you can balance your cortisol levels while boosting production of leptin, a type of hormone that causes you to control your appetite.

Dining Late at Night

Eating late and sleeping on a full stomach increases your risk of developing acid reflux and indigestion, since gravity is no longer able to pull down everything in your stomach. To prevent these conditions, consider eating smaller meals at night and don't lie down for at least three hours after dinner. If possible, just snack on fruits in case you feel a bit hungry at night instead of raiding the fridge for sweet desserts to satisfy your craving.

Foods to Avoid

Wheat
Wheat is the result of 40 years of genetics research aimed to increase yield-per-acre. The result is a genetically-unique plant that stands 18-24 inches tall, and not the natural flowing fields of 4 1/2-foot tall "amber waves of grain" we all remember.

Wheat contains gluten which triggers a host of immune diseases like celiac, rheumatoid arthritis, and gluten encephalopathy (dementia from wheat). Gladden, the protein unique to wheat, is odd in that it is weakened in the human gastrointestinal tract to peptides (small proteins) that have the ability to cross into the brain and bind to morphine receptors.

When you remove wheat from the diet, you've removed the gliadin protein which leads to the stimulation of appetite, and so your appetite and craving to eat drops. The average daily calorie intake drops 400 calories per day with less hunger, less cravings and food is more satisfying. This all occurs without imposing calorie limits, cutting fat grams, or limiting portion size. It all happens just by eliminating wheat.

Wheat free and gluten free alternative flours are Amaranth flour, Banana flour, Arrowroot flour and Brown rice flour and many more.

Carbs
The reduced-carb diet promoted the loss of visceral fat even when no change in weight was apparent.

Visceral fat is strongly linked with type 2 diabetes, heart disease, stroke, and other chronic diseases. It is thought that visceral fat is related to the release of proteins and hormones that can cause inflammation, which in turn can damage arteries and enter your liver, affecting how your body breaks down sugars and fats.

While it's often referred to as "belly fat" because it can cause a "beer belly" or an apple-shaped body, you can have visceral fat even if you're thin. So even if you aren't trying to lose weight, cutting unhealthy carbs in your diet could have a positive impact on your levels of visceral fat, and thereby potentially reduce your risk of chronic disease.

Many people resist the idea of cutting grain and sugar from their diets, wondering what else there is to eat if they avoid bread, potatoes, pizza, baked goods and other unhealthy carbs.

Slow-release carbohydrates are low on the glycemic index. These carbs are good for keeping blood sugar stable. The higher a food's score on the glycemic index, the quicker it raises blood sugar. Low glycemic foods include red lentils, baked beans, apples, lentils, peas, peanuts, grapefruit, cherries, dried apricots, green beans, butter beans, chickpeas, kidney beans and navy beans.

Soda drink
On average, a can of non-diet cola contains about 135 calories. If you drink three cans a day, you're getting roughly 405 daily calories from soft drinks. A pound of fat equals 3,500 calories, so if all other things in your diet are equal, cutting out soda spares you more than a pound of fat every 10 days. Plus, soda lacks significant levels of any essential vitamins or minerals. All soda contributes to your diet is sugar, and those calories are much better spent on foods with higher nutritional value.

Refines Sugar
Refined sugar helps to raise the insulin level in the body which promotes the storage of fat. It also affects the immune system and makes it harder to fight off germs and diseases. Sugar has the potential to make you fat.

Sugar hides behind many names such as dextrose, corn syrup, corn sweetener, high fructose corn syrup, glucose, fruit juice concentrate, honey, lactose, maltose, sucrose, malt syrup and molasses. The American Heart Association (AHA) indicates that the average American gets an inordinate amount of sugar each day (more than 22 teaspoons, or around 355 calories). When you consume more calories than you burn each day, the excess is stored in your body in the form of fat, which shows around the belly as well as other areas.

Foods that Fight Belly Fat

Omega-3 fatty acids

If you have constant chronic inflammation, you'll have a very difficult time losing weight. In fact, some experts believe it's impossible to lose excessive belly fat without addressing chronic inflammation. There are a lot of foods that fight inflammation, but foods rich in omega-3s are the very best as they help to reduce cortisol levels.

Research has shown that a diet with a high percentage of omega-3 fatty acids and a low percentage of omega-6 fatty acids has been linked with decreased inflammation. Food sources of omega-3s include walnuts, flaxseed, and fish, such as wild Alaskan salmon.

Spices
Certain spices including garlic, turmeric, cinnamon, ginger, and chili peppers, have potent inflammation-reducing capabilities, so try adding them to meals as often as possible.

Water
Staying hydrated is essential to flushing inflammation-causing toxins out of your body. Aim for 64 ounces of water per day. When exercising, it is important to remember to drink an additional 8 ounces of water for every 30 minutes to replenish what the body has sweated out.

Lemon Water
The connection between our liver and belly fat may not be immediately apparent, but they are indeed related. Our liver is a powerhouse of an organ that can take a beating, but like an air filter, the liver can get clogged up if it's not maintained and cleaned. Lemon water helps to do that. As our liver secretes bile to break down fat, the lemon water can help to thin out the bile and keep toxins flowing

through your liver, then out of your body. As a result, fat metabolism becomes more optimal.

Juice one lemon, or simply add about two tablespoons of lemon juice to one cup of warm water. Drink every morning before you eat to give your liver a helping hand.

Fruits and vegetables

A 2014 study published on obesity looked at the diets of more than 400,000 adults in America, and found that less than 4 percent of adults actually ate 9 serving of fruits and vegetables daily. More than three-quarters of U.S. adults get fewer than 5 servings per day. The same study also found that eating fruits and vegetables was linked with better weight control, even without other factors that can help weight loss. So simply including fruits and vegetables is a major advantage to burning belly fat.

Green tea

People in Asia have been drinking green tea daily and have reaped the rewards of improved resistance to disease, low joint pain, enhanced cardiovascular function and flat bellies.

Green tea is rich in a special fat-burning compound called EGCG (epigallocatechin gallate). This catechin has been shown in cellular studies to prevent the growth and differentiation of adipocytes (fat cells), which is how and why belly fat occurs in the first place.

In a study published in "The American Journal of Clinical Nutrition" in 2010, researchers analyzed results from 15 trials involving the effects of green tea on weight and body composition. They found that subjects who consumed green-tea catechins with caffeine saw a greater decrease in waist circumference and weight loss, than those who only consumed caffeine. A smaller waistline generally indicates a smaller stomach, so these results show promise if you're aiming for a flatter stomach.

Monounsaturated Fats
Monounsaturated fats added to a balanced diet will help promote fat loss through your midsection.

The March 2007 issue of the "Journal For Diabetes Care" explained that eating a source of monounsaturated fatty acids with each meal of your day will help your body burn fat from the stomach area. Monounsaturated fats help to increase your basal metabolic rate allowing your body to burn fat. Some favorite sources of monounsaturated fats include: Olives, Olive oil, Peanuts, Macadamia nuts, Hazelnuts and Avocados.

Apple Cider Vinegar

A shot of apple cider vinegar once a day might be just what you need to get your body moving in the right direction. It contains a host of vitamins, minerals and acetic acid. Acetic acid is what makes ACV shine by controlling appetite, increasing insulin sensitivity (a good thing), and helping to produce protein in the body that helps decrease fat storage. Another great benefit of apple cider vinegar is that it helps to make the blood more alkaline. Our body's pH level should be slightly alkaline, but unhealthy foods and stress create a more acidic environment.

Only buy unfiltered apple cider vinegar to get the greatest benefit. Filtered vinegar doesn't have the same effect.

Nutrients that shrink your Belly

Methylhydroxy chalcone polymer (MHCP) in Cinnamon

MHCP is an active compound found in cinnamon which makes fat cells more receptive to insulin.

When cells are more receptive to insulin, they allow the insulin to transport sugar into the cells for energy, thus keeping insulin levels in the bloodstream low. High insulin levels trigger the body to store more fat, especially in your midsection. So consuming a seasoning like cinnamon that helps maintain healthy levels of insulin is a great way to combat belly fat.

Caraway Seeds

Bloating and gas can occur in your gastrointestinal tract for a number of reasons. Caraway seeds are effective at reducing gas and bloating because they're a powerful digestive aid. They help to expel and eliminate gas due to their carminative properties. Caraway seeds are also beneficial at keeping bloatedness away because they help the good bacteria in your gastrointestinal tract digest and break down food while inhibiting the growth of the bad bacteria.

Fucoxanthin

Research on this compound suggests it may be a powerful fat fighter. In animal studies, overweight and obese mice were found to lose 5 to 10 percent of their entire body weight when consuming fucoxanthin. Although research is still unclear as to exactly how fucoxanthin promotes weight loss, it may be due to its ability to target a specific protein that increases the rate at which abdominal fat is burned. Edible brown seaweed is available in Japanese specialty stores and health food stores under the names *wakame* and *hijiki*.

Quercetin

Quercetin is a flavonoid effective at decreasing inflammation in the body as well as blocking baby fat cells from maturing and is more effective at inhibiting the rate of new fat cell formation than any other flavonoid. Large amounts of quercetin are found in apples, onions (especially red onions), and green tea. Red grapes, tomatoes, broccoli, cherries, raspberries, and leafy greens are also excellent sources. Aim to take in quercetin from foods rather than supplements, because foods rich in quercetin contain many additional health benefits.

Resveratrol

Resveratrol has also been shown to suppress levels of the hormone estrogen. High levels of estrogen in your body promote increased fat storage, so suppressing these levels may decrease body fat while helping to increase lean muscle mass. Resveratrol is found in red grapes, red wine, peanuts, and dark chocolate.

Vitamin C

Vitamin C helps to reduce the stress hormone cortisol to normal levels after a stressful situation. This reduction in cortisol may also help to prevent increased belly-fat storage.

Aim to consume at least two foods rich in vitamin C each day. Options include oranges, kiwis, and green peppers. Vitamin C is available in supplement form, but taking in nutrients through food is always the best option. If you do opt for a supplement, keep your dosage to 500 milligrams per day and choose a time-released formula for the best benefit.

Calcium Pyruvate
Calcium Pyruvate occurs naturally in the body during digestion and metabolism to make energy and fuel your cells.

A study done by the University of Pittsburgh found that obese women lost 48 percent more fat when following a calorie-restricted diet with supplemental calcium pyruvate than those women following the diet alone. It appears that calcium pyruvate can get into the fat cells and help them burn energy more effectively, promoting more weight loss.

Smoothies

Smoothie diets have become popular way to introduce healthier food to the body with the intention of burning fat. Most popular as a breakfast option, substituting another meal for lunch or dinner is perfectly acceptable. A smoothie is also a great choice for an after workout snack.

Green smoothies can end up as belly fat, but only if you don't balance the calories they contain with the rest of your food intake as well as an exercise routine. Too many calories, too little exercise, muscle loss and hormonal changes cause belly fat, not one specific food. That means you can enjoy your blender concoctions as long as you account for the calories they contain and adjust accordingly.

The Surprising Number of Calories in a Smoothie
If you toss some green vegetables, yogurt, milk, a banana, protein powder and some wheat germ into your blender, your 2- to-3 cup smoothie will contain well over 500 calories. If you add additional fruits, nuts, peanut butter, chocolate sauce, flax seeds, healthy fats or sweeteners, your calorie tally goes even higher.

Making a Lighter Smoothie

Small changes to your smoothie recipe can cut your calories in half. For example, you can switch from whole milk, which has 150 calories per cup, to fat-free milk, which has only 90. Opt for fat-free yogurt instead of full-fat and use extra fruit instead of sugar or other sweeteners. The U.S. Centers for Disease Control and Prevention recommends ordering a child-sized smoothie if you don't make the drink at home.

Balanced Smoothie Intake

If you weigh 155 pounds and you down a 500-calorie smoothie for breakfast, you can burn off those calories playing basketball, running at 2 miles per hour or cycling at 12 miles per hour for 60 minutes. If you run at a fast pace, such as 8 miles per hour, play soccer or cycle faster than 20 miles per hour, you can burn that smoothie off in just 30 minutes. You can also reduce the number of calories from your daily meals and snacks so that, even if you have a 500 calorie smoothie, you still only take in the number of calories you need to maintain your weight or lose weight. Again, it is about a combination of calorie control and exercise usually works best at fighting belly fat.

Smoothie Recipes

Flat-Belly Smoothie

This deliciously sweet smoothie is packed with ingredients to fight belly fat and reduce bloating, and comes in at under 300 calories. The Greek yogurt in the recipe provides a good amount of calcium and protein, both of which can aid in weight loss. Pineapple contains an enzyme that helps ease digestion and banish bloat. Kale is full of fiber to prevent constipation, and water to help cleanse.

Ingredients

3 ounces vanilla nonfat Greek yogurt

1 tablespoon almond butter

1/2 cup frozen blueberries

1/2 cup frozen pineapple

1 cup kale

3/4 cup water

Directions

Place all the ingredients in a blender, and mix until smooth.

Berries Smoothie

Berries are nutritional all-stars that should have a special part in your weight loss plan. They are low in calories and high in water and antioxidants so they help your body get rid of extra weight, lose belly fat and reduce cellulite.

Recent researches state that people who consume food rich in antioxidants weigh less irrespective of the number of calories taken. Antioxidants boost metabolism, suppress appetite and reduce sugar cravings.

Ingredients
1/2 cup raspberries (fresh or frozen)

1/4 cup blueberries

1/4 cup blackberries

1/2 apple

1/2 banana

1/3 cup fresh orange juice

Instructions
Combine the ingredients and process well till smooth and creamy. Enjoy.

Mango and Pineapple Smoothie
Mango and pineapple are great advantage for all those wanting to lose weight. They act as a natural fat burning foods so implementing them into your diet will certainly help you lose weight with visible results. Loaded with fiber, the most vital weight loss ingredient, they aid digestion, boost metabolism and speed up the process of melting excess fat in the body.

Ingredients

1 cup chopped mango

1/2 cup pineapple chunks

1/4 cup apple juice

1 tbsp flax seeds

Instructions

Put the ingredients in a blend and blend for short till you get creamy smoothie with rich texture.

Kiwi Smoothie

Kiwi are packed with weight loss promoting compounds and are really an excellent idea for all those who want to win the battle over extra pounds. They are rich in fiber and low in glycemic index and help you feel full for longer thus preventing consumption of extra food and calories.

Ingredients

4 kiwifruits

1 banana

a handful of spinach

1/4 cup fresh lemon juice

Instructions

Mix the listed ingredients and blend for a minute till everything goes smooth and silky. Enjoy the delicious and refreshing drink.

Breakfast Smoothies

Skipping breakfast will slow your metabolism and leave you hungry by lunch. Instead, start your day with the one meal that can beat bloat while helping to flatten your stomach, stabilize your blood sugar, and jump-start your body's fat-burning powers. Start your day the right way with the morning smoothie.

Blue Ginger Smoothie

This phytonutrient-filled, omega-3-rich smoothie will help you start your day off right with a burst of raw, green energy.

Ingredients

2 cups almond milk or coconut-almond milk

½ English cucumber

1 cup baby spinach

1 cup Swiss chard

1 tablespoon almond butter

5 walnut halves

1 teaspoon vanilla extract

1 teaspoon spirulina

3-4 tablespoons (approx. 37.5-50 grams) protein powder

⅛ teaspoon sea salt

⅛ teaspoon cinnamon

¼ cup ice (2 cubes from an ice cube tray), optional

Directions
Add all the ingredients in the order given to the blender.
Blend until smooth

Blue Ginger Smoothie
Rich in minerals and phytonutrients, this smoothie features an antioxidant-rich blue-green algae called chlorella. Along with that it also contains tasty blueberries, ginger, and Brazil nuts. It is super-charged for healthier digestion while helping improve hair and skin.

Ingredients
1 cup frozen blueberries

¼ cup whole Brazil nuts

1½ cups filtered water

2 teaspoon chlorella (in powder form)

1 large handful spinach

One 2-inch piece ginger (about 1 tbsp), peeled and finely grated

1 tablespoon coconut oil

3-4 tablespoons (approx. 37.5-50 grams) protein powder

¼ cup almond milk (optional; add for a creamier finish)

1 sprig of mint leaves (optional)

Directions
Add all the ingredients in the order given to the blender. Blend until smooth.

Goji- Strawberry Smoothie
Powered by goji berries and the soothing flavor of coconut manna, this strawberry-enhanced smoothie will please your taste buds while keeping you full and happy for hours.

Ingredients
¼ cup fresh or frozen organic strawberries

1 cup almond milk

¼ cup filtered water

¼ cup coconut water

1-2 tablespoons goji powder

1 tablespoon coconut manna

3-4 tablespoons (approx. 37.5-50 grams) protein powder

Ice cubes (optional)

Goji berries (optional; for garnish)

Directions
1. Freeze fresh strawberries the night before.

2. Place all ingredients in a high-speed blender and blend until smooth.

3. Add a few ice cubes if you prefer a cooler, thicker smoothie.

4. Enjoy with a garnish of goji berries.

Chocolate – Covered Almond Smoothie

The secret ingredient in this smoothie is hemp hearts, or shelled seeds of the hemp plant that are rich in difficult-to-find omega-3 fatty acids, along with protein, vitamins, and healthy enzymes.

Ingredients

2 cups almond milk or coconut-almond milk

2 teaspoons cacao powder

2 tablespoons almond butter

1 teaspoon vanilla extract

1 teaspoon ground chia seeds

1/4 teaspoon ground nutmeg

3-4 tablespoons (approx. 37.5-50 grams) protein powder

1/4 cup hemp hearts

Directions

Add all the ingredients in the order given to the blender. Blend until smooth.

The 5:2 fast Diet

The Fast Diet, is currently the most popular intermittent fasting diet out there because many people find the Fast Diets way of eating to be easier to stick to than a traditional calorie-restricted diet. It's called the 5:2 diet because five days of the week are normal eating days, while the other two restrict calories to 500 for women 600 for men per day. Since you are only fasting for two days of your choice each week, and eating normally on the other five days, there is always something new and tasty on the near horizon. It is easier easy to comply with a regime that only asks you to restrict your calorie intake occasionally, rather than a complete overhaul of diet. It recalibrates the diet equation, and stacks the odds in your favor. It is more of an eating pattern than a diet. There are no requirements about the foods you eat, but rather when you should eat them.

How to Apply the 5:2 Diet
The 5:2 diet is very simple: For five days a week you eat as you normally would without worrying about restricting calories. On the other two days you reduce your calorie intake to a quarter of your daily needs. This is about 500 calories per day for women, and 600 for men.

You can choose the two days of the week you prefer, as long as there is at least 1 non-fasting day in between. The 5:2 diet is very effective for weight loss, if done correctly. It will help reduce belly fat, as well as help maintain muscle mass during weight loss.

How to Eat on Fasting Days
There is no rule as to what or when you must eat on the fasting days. Some people function best by beginning the day with a small breakfast, while others find it best to start eating as late as possible.

Generally, there are two meal patterns that people use:

Three small meals: Usually breakfast, lunch and dinner.

Two slightly bigger meals: Only lunch and dinner.

Since calorie intake is limited — 500 for women and 600 for men — it makes sense to use your calorie budget wisely.

Here are some examples of suitable fast day foods:

- Natural yogurt with berries.
- Boiled or baked eggs.
- A generous portion of vegetables.
- Soups (for example miso, tomato, cauliflower or vegetable).
- Low-calorie cup soups.

- Grilled fish or lean meat.
- Cauliflower rice.
- Black coffee.
- Tea.
- Still or sparkling water

Exercises to do

The ultimate way to achieve a toned, flat tummy is to combine a healthy diet like the Fast Diet with aerobic exercise. Here are some very effective routines.

The Roll-Up
Hold a resistance band taut between your hands and lie on the floor face up, with legs extended and arms overhead. Pull abs in, tuck your chin, lift arms toward the ceiling, and roll head, shoulders, and torso up and over your legs as far as you can. Keep heels firmly on the floor and reach hands towards your feet. Pause, then slowly roll back down. Do 5 to 8 reps with 30 minutes of cardio 5 to 6 times a week.

The Spiderman Climber
Get into plank position with arms and legs extended, hands beneath shoulders, and feet flexed. Keeping your abs tight, bend your left leg out to the side and bring the knee toward the left elbow. Pause, then return to start. Switch sides. Do 20 reps, alternating sides, with 30 minutes of cardio 5 to 6 times a week.

Talk and walk

A weekly walk-and-talk session with an exercise buddy is an easy social solution to getting some aerobic exercise. With a friend you can take a walk around your city, form a friendly fitness club, or try a new class at the gym together.

Cardio

If you want to burn the most belly fat, a Duke University study confirms that aerobic exercise is the most effective in burning that deep, visceral belly fat. In fact, aerobic training burns 67% more calories than resistance training or a combination of the two, according to the study.

The Windshield Wiper

Lie face-up with arms out to your sides, palms down, and legs bent at 90 degrees so feet are off the floor. Keep abs tight and slowly lower legs to the left as far as possible, keeping shoulders on the floor. Pause, then return to start. Repeat to the right. Do 20 reps, alternating sides.

Household Chores

Something which goes unnoticed is the possibility of exercising whilst cleaning the house. Vacuuming is a great ab workout. Tighten your abdominal muscles while you push back and forth for a tighter tummy while you clean.

Boxing

Take your workout indoors with boxing. Aerobic kickboxing is more than just a great belly fat-burning, cardio workout. All those arm thrusts and high kicks firm abs, too.

Try Playing Catch

Lie on your back, knees bent, feet flat on the floor, shoulders and head off the floor with your abs contracted. Then have someone throw an exercise ball (or a basketball) to you. Alternate between your left and right side so you have to twist and reach to catch it. Do this as many times as is comfortable, and try to increase the number each week.

Try Sitting

While you're driving, sitting, or just waiting at the doctor's office, imagine there's gum or wet paint on the back of your chair so you have to hold yourself up instead of leaning back. Keep shoulder blades down and back, abdominals lifted, and picture yourself knitting your rib cage together and in.

Conclusion to Belly Fat

The unhealthy dangers of belly fat should be enough reason to work toward a flat stomach. Study after study have shown that the people with larger waist sizes have the highest risk of life-threatening disease. According to the National Institutes of Health, a waistline larger than 40 inches for men and 35 inches for women signals significant risk of heart disease and diabetes. The evidence couldn't be more convincing.

By simply losing body fat you can improve your sex life from building strong abdominal and lower-back muscles for improved stamina and strength for try new positions, so that sex is as pleasurable as it should be.

Most back pain is related to weak muscles in the trunk of your body, so maintaining a strong midsection can help resolve many back issues. The muscles that crisscross your midsection don't function in isolation; they weave through your torso like a spiderweb, even attaching to your spine. When your abdominal muscles are weak, the muscles in your butt and along the backs of your legs have to compensate for the work your abs should be doing

Having a big belly and a fatty neck can trigger chronic, loud snoring and its partner, a sleep disorder called sleep apnea. People who have sleep apnea literally stop breathing for a few seconds to more than a minute hundreds of times a night, disrupting their sleep. As a result they end up feeling exhausted the next morning and lack energy to concentrate and make important decisions. Losing weight can often help remedy the problem so you can get a better night's sleep.

A bulge in the belly is a wake-up call. If you can trim down your midsection, you'll go a long way toward preventing the health problems associated with belly fat. A healthy lifestyle can ward off fat from top to bottom, and especially the middle. When you lose weight, your body will make getting rid of belly fat its top priority. If you manage to lose just 5 to 10 percent of your overall body weight, you can reduce the hazardous layer of belly fat by as much as 30 percent.

Reference

http://www.getprograde.com/green-tea-and-belly-fat.html

http://www.shape.com/weight-loss/tips-plans/ask-diet-doctor-fat-burning-foods

http://www.prevention.com/weight-loss/weight-loss-tips/tips-flat-belly

http://www.womenshealthmag.com/weight-loss/eliminate-belly-fat-0

http://www.livestrong.com/article/458796-fruits-vegetables-that-burn-belly-fat/

www.ingramcontent.com/pod-product-compliance
Lightning Source LLC
Chambersburg PA
CBHW071313280526
45788CB00004B/1890